My Essential Oil Recipes

a blank recipe book for <u>your</u> recipes & records

Thank you for your purchase!

This blank recipe book is intended as place to record your blends of oils and keep recipes you love from all other places.
You will also notice that there are areas to record each family members results to the recipe. This is great for reference.

At the back of the book you will find a list of essential oils.
I hope this helps you track your inventory.

Recipe Index

pg	Recipe	Condition	Diffuse	External	Internal
10					
11					
12					
13					
14					
15					
16					
17					
18					
19					
20					
21					
22					
23					
24					
25					
26					

pg	Recipe	Condition	🌀	🧴	👤
27					
28					
29					
30					
31					
34					
35					
36					
37					
38					
39					
40					
41					
42					
43					
44					
45					
46					

pg	Recipe	Condition	〽	🖐	👤
47					
48					
49					
50					
51					
54					
55					
56					
57					
58					
59					
60					
61					
62					
63					
64					
65					
66					

pg	Recipe	Condition	༄	💧	👤
67					
68					
69					
70					
71					
74					
75					
76					
77					
78					
79					
80					
81					
82					
83					
84					
85					
86					

pg	Recipe	Condition	ꝿꝉ	🖐️	👤
87					
88					
89					
90					
91					
94					
95					
96					
97					
98					
99					
100					
101					
102					
103					
104					
105					
106					

pg	Recipe	Condition	ᛦ	✋	🗣
107					
108					
109	.				
110					
111					
114					
115					
116					
117					
118					
119					
120					
121					
122					
123					
124					
125					
126					

pg	Recipe	Condition	〰	💧	👤
127					
128					
129					
130					
131					
134					
135					
136					
137					
138					
139					
140					
141					
142					
143					
144					
145					
146					

pg	Recipe	Condition	ᛝ	💧	🗣
147					

How to fill in a Recipe (Sample)

Recipe Name: Lavender & Citrus Freshener ᛝ 💧 🗣

1 tsp	vodka
15 drops	lavender essential oil
10 drops	grapefruit essential oil
500 ml	water

Uses: Mix together the vodka and essential oils in a 500ml spray bottle and shake well. Add water and shake again. Spray a fine mist into the air. Avoid spraying directly on fabrics or wood surfaces.

Family Results Record:

Date	Family Member	Condition	Application	Result
24 Apr	Joey	hyper	air	calming

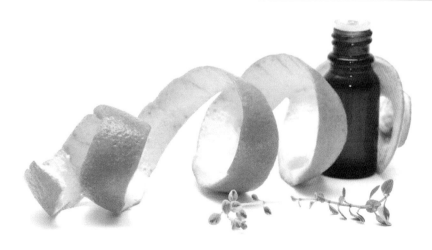

Recipe Name:

Uses:

Family Results Record:

Date	Family Member	Condition	Application	Result

Recipe Name:

Uses:

Family Results Record:

Date	Family Member	Condition	Application	Result

Recipe Name:

Uses:

Family Results Record:

Date	Family Member	Condition	Application	Result

Recipe Name:

Uses:

Family Results Record:

Date	Family Member	Condition	Application	Result

Recipe Name:

Uses:

Family Results Record:

Date	Family Member	Condition	Application	Result

Recipe Name:

Uses:

Family Results Record:

Date	Family Member	Condition	Application	Result

Recipe Name:

Uses:

Family Results Record:

Date	Family Member	Condition	Application	Result

Recipe Name:

Uses:

Family Results Record:

Date	Family Member	Condition	Application	Result

Recipe Name:

Uses:

Family Results Record:

Date	Family Member	Condition	Application	Result

Recipe Name:

Uses:

Family Results Record:

Date	Family Member	Condition	Application	Result

Recipe Name:

Uses:

Family Results Record:

Date	Family Member	Condition	Application	Result

Recipe Name:

Uses:

Family Results Record:

Date	Family Member	Condition	Application	Result

Recipe Name:

Uses:

Family Results Record:

Date	Family Member	Condition	Application	Result

Recipe Name:

Uses:

Family Results Record:

Date	Family Member	Condition	Application	Result

Recipe Name:

Uses:

Family Results Record:

Date	Family Member	Condition	Application	Result

Recipe Name:

Uses:

Family Results Record:

Date	Family Member	Condition	Application	Result

Recipe Name:

Uses:

Family Results Record:

Date	Family Member	Condition	Application	Result

Recipe Name:

Uses:

Family Results Record:

Date	Family Member	Condition	Application	Result

Recipe Name:

Uses:

Family Results Record:

Date	Family Member	Condition	Application	Result

Recipe Name:

Uses:

Family Results Record:

Date	Family Member	Condition	Application	Result

Recipe Name:

Uses:

Family Results Record:

Date	Family Member	Condition	Application	Result

Recipe Name:

Uses:

Family Results Record:

Date	Family Member	Condition	Application	Result

Recipe Name:

Uses:

Family Results Record:

Date	Family Member	Condition	Application	Result

Recipe Name:

Uses:

Family Results Record:

Date	Family Member	Condition	Application	Result

Recipe Name:

Uses:

Family Results Record:

Date	Family Member	Condition	Application	Result

Recipe Name:

Uses:

Family Results Record:

Date	Family Member	Condition	Application	Result

Recipe Name:

Uses:

Family Results Record:

Date	Family Member	Condition	Application	Result

Recipe Name:

Uses:

Family Results Record:

Date	Family Member	Condition	Application	Result

Recipe Name:

Uses:

Family Results Record:

Date	Family Member	Condition	Application	Result

Recipe Name:

Uses:

Family Results Record:

Date	Family Member	Condition	Application	Result

Recipe Name:

Uses:

Family Results Record:

Date	Family Member	Condition	Application	Result

Recipe Name:

Uses:

Family Results Record:

Date	Family Member	Condition	Application	Result

Recipe Name:

Uses:

Family Results Record:

Date	Family Member	Condition	Application	Result

Recipe Name:

Uses:

Family Results Record:

Date	Family Member	Condition	Application	Result

Recipe Name:

Uses:

Family Results Record:

Date	Family Member	Condition	Application	Result

Recipe Name:

Uses:

Family Results Record:

Date	Family Member	Condition	Application	Result

Recipe Name:

Uses:

Family Results Record:

Date	Family Member	Condition	Application	Result

Recipe Name:

Uses:

Family Results Record:

Date	Family Member	Condition	Application	Result

Recipe Name:

Uses:

Family Results Record:

Date	Family Member	Condition	Application	Result

Recipe Name:

Uses:

Family Results Record:

Date	Family Member	Condition	Application	Result

Recipe Name:

Uses:

Family Results Record:

Date	Family Member	Condition	Application	Result

Recipe Name:

Uses:

Family Results Record:

Date	Family Member	Condition	Application	Result

Recipe Name:

Uses:

Family Results Record:

Date	Family Member	Condition	Application	Result

Recipe Name:

Uses:

Family Results Record:

Date	Family Member	Condition	Application	Result

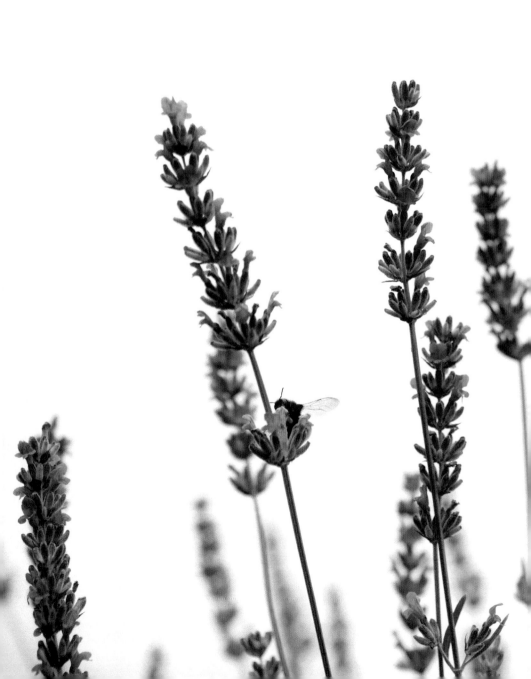

Lavender

allergies
insomnia
anxiety
cold sores
burns
dandruff
yeast infections
ringworm
rash
and more

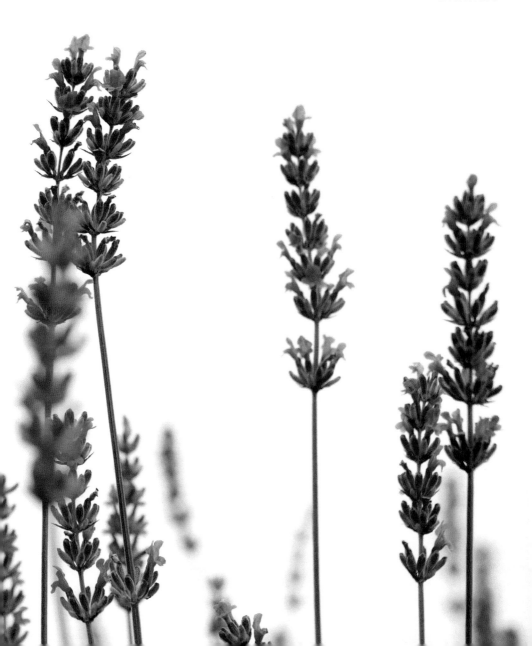

Recipe Name:

Uses:

Family Results Record:

Date	Family Member	Condition	Application	Result

Recipe Name:

Uses:

Family Results Record:

Date	Family Member	Condition	Application	Result

Recipe Name:

Uses:

Family Results Record:

Date	Family Member	Condition	Application	Result

Recipe Name:

Uses:

Family Results Record:

Date	Family Member	Condition	Application	Result

Recipe Name:

Uses:

Family Results Record:

Date	Family Member	Condition	Application	Result

Recipe Name:

Uses:

Family Results Record:

Date	Family Member	Condition	Application	Result

Recipe Name:

Uses:

Family Results Record:

Date	Family Member	Condition	Application	Result

Recipe Name:

Uses:

Family Results Record:

Date	Family Member	Condition	Application	Result

Recipe Name:

Uses:

Family Results Record:

Date	Family Member	Condition	Application	Result

Recipe Name:

Uses:

Family Results Record:

Date	Family Member	Condition	Application	Result

Recipe Name:

Uses:

Family Results Record:

Date	Family Member	Condition	Application	Result

Recipe Name:

Uses:

Family Results Record:

Date	Family Member	Condition	Application	Result

Recipe Name:

Uses:

Family Results Record:

Date	Family Member	Condition	Application	Result

Recipe Name:

Uses:

Family Results Record:

Date	Family Member	Condition	Application	Result

Recipe Name:

Uses:

Family Results Record:

Date	Family Member	Condition	Application	Result

Recipe Name:

Uses:

Family Results Record:

Date	Family Member	Condition	Application	Result

Recipe Name:

Uses:

Family Results Record:

Date	Family Member	Condition	Application	Result
				.

Recipe Name:

Uses:

Family Results Record:

Date	Family Member	Condition	Application	Result

Recipe Name:

Uses:

Family Results Record:

Date	Family Member	Condition	Application	Result

Recipe Name:

Uses:

Family Results Record:

Date	Family Member	Condition	Application	Result

Recipe Name:

Uses:

Family Results Record:

Date	Family Member	Condition	Application	Result

Recipe Name:

Uses:

Family Results Record:

Date	Family Member	Condition	Application	Result

Recipe Name:

Uses:

Family Results Record:

Date	Family Member	Condition	Application	Result

Recipe Name:

Uses:

Family Results Record:

Date	Family Member	Condition	Application	Result

Recipe Name:

Uses:

Family Results Record:

Date	Family Member	Condition	Application	Result

Recipe Name:

Uses:

Family Results Record:

Date	Family Member	Condition	Application	Result

Recipe Name:

Uses:

Family Results Record:

Date	Family Member	Condition	Application	Result

Recipe Name:

Uses:

Family Results Record:

Date	Family Member	Condition	Application	Result

Recipe Name:

Uses:

Family Results Record:

Date	Family Member	Condition	Application	Result

Recipe Name:

Uses:

Family Results Record:

Date	Family Member	Condition	Application	Result

Recipe Name:

Uses:

Family Results Record:

Date	Family Member	Condition	Application	Result

Recipe Name:

Uses:

Family Results Record:

Date	Family Member	Condition	Application	Result

Recipe Name:

Uses:

Family Results Record:

Date	Family Member	Condition	Application	Result

Recipe Name:

Uses:

Family Results Record:

Date	Family Member	Condition	Application	Result

Recipe Name:

Uses:

Family Results Record:

Date	Family Member	Condition	Application	Result

Recipe Name:

Uses:

Family Results Record:

Date	Family Member	Condition	Application	Result

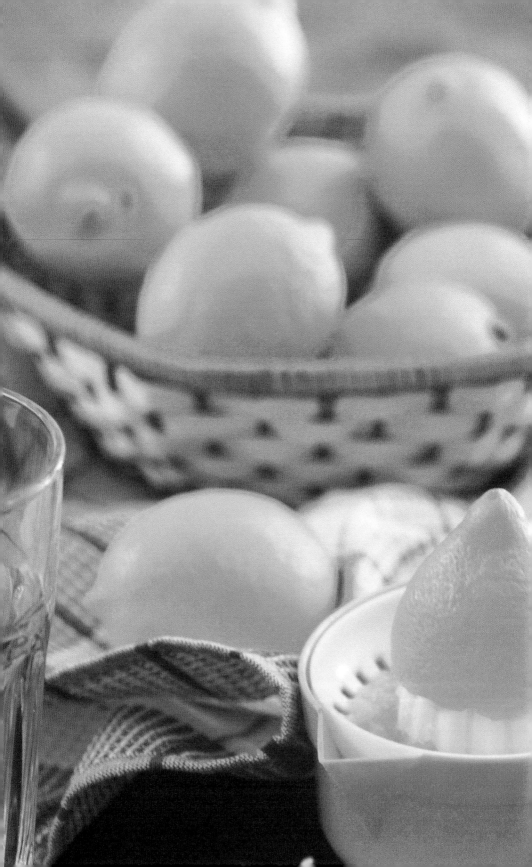

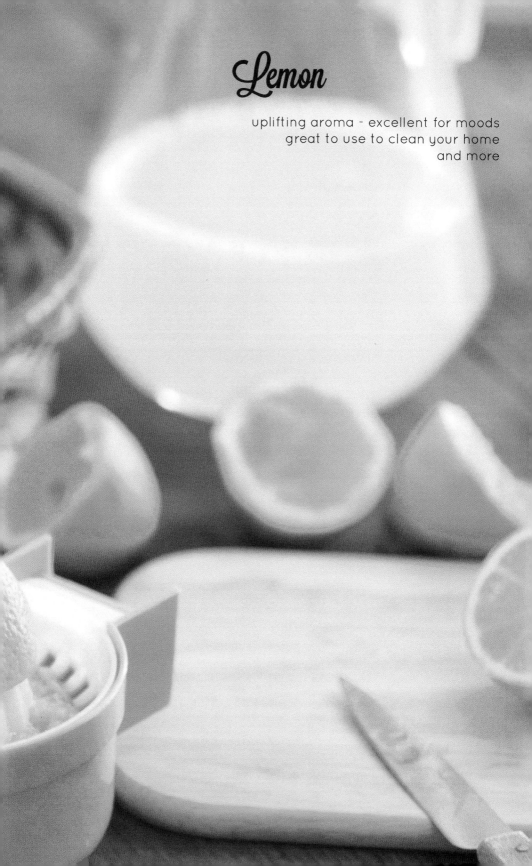

Lemon

uplifting aroma - excellent for moods
great to use to clean your home
and more

Recipe Name:

Uses:

Family Results Record:

Date	Family Member	Condition	Application	Result

Recipe Name:

Uses:

Family Results Record:

Date	Family Member	Condition	Application	Result

Recipe Name:

Uses:

Family Results Record:

Date	Family Member	Condition	Application	Result

Recipe Name:

Uses:

Family Results Record:

Date	Family Member	Condition	Application	Result

Recipe Name:

Uses:

Family Results Record:

Date	Family Member	Condition	Application	Result

Recipe Name:

Uses:

Family Results Record:

Date	Family Member	Condition	Application	Result

Recipe Name:

Uses:

Family Results Record:

Date	Family Member	Condition	Application	Result

Recipe Name:

Uses:

Family Results Record:

Date	Family Member	Condition	Application	Result

Recipe Name:

Uses:

Family Results Record:

Date	Family Member	Condition	Application	Result

Recipe Name:

Uses:

Family Results Record:

Date	Family Member	Condition	Application	Result

Recipe Name:

Uses:

Family Results Record:

Date	Family Member	Condition	Application	Result

Recipe Name:

Uses:

Family Results Record:

Date	Family Member	Condition	Application	Result

Recipe Name:

Uses:

Family Results Record:

Date	Family Member	Condition	Application	Result

Recipe Name:

Uses:

Family Results Record:

Date	Family Member	Condition	Application	Result

Recipe Name:

Uses:

Family Results Record:

Date	Family Member	Condition	Application	Result

Recipe Name:

Uses:

Family Results Record:

Date	Family Member	Condition	Application	Result

Recipe Name:

Uses:

Family Results Record:

Date	Family Member	Condition	Application	Result

Recipe Name:

Uses:

Family Results Record:

Date	Family Member	Condition	Application	Result

Recipe Name:

Uses:

Family Results Record:

Date	Family Member	Condition	Application	Result

Recipe Name:

Uses:

Family Results Record:

Date	Family Member	Condition	Application	Result

Recipe Name:

Uses:

Family Results Record:

Date	Family Member	Condition	Application	Result

Recipe Name:

Uses:

Family Results Record:

Date	Family Member	Condition	Application	Result

Recipe Name:

Uses:

Family Results Record:

Date	Family Member	Condition	Application	Result

Recipe Name:

Uses:

Family Results Record:

Date	Family Member	Condition	Application	Result

Recipe Name:

Uses:

Family Results Record:

Date	Family Member	Condition	Application	Result

Recipe Name:

Uses:

Family Results Record:

Date	Family Member	Condition	Application	Result

Recipe Name:

Uses:

Family Results Record:

Date	Family Member	Condition	Application	Result

Recipe Name:

Uses:

Family Results Record:

Date	Family Member	Condition	Application	Result

Recipe Name:

Uses:

Family Results Record:

Date	Family Member	Condition	Application	Result

Recipe Name:

Uses:

Family Results Record:

Date	Family Member	Condition	Application	Result

Recipe Name:

Uses:

Family Results Record:

Date	Family Member	Condition	Application	Result

Recipe Name:

Uses:

Family Results Record:

Date	Family Member	Condition	Application	Result

Recipe Name:

Uses:

Family Results Record:

Date	Family Member	Condition	Application	Result

Recipe Name:

Uses:

Family Results Record:

Date	Family Member	Condition	Application	Result

Recipe Name:

Uses:

Family Results Record:

Date	Family Member	Condition	Application	Result

Recipe Name:

Uses:

Family Results Record:

Date	Family Member	Condition	Application	Result

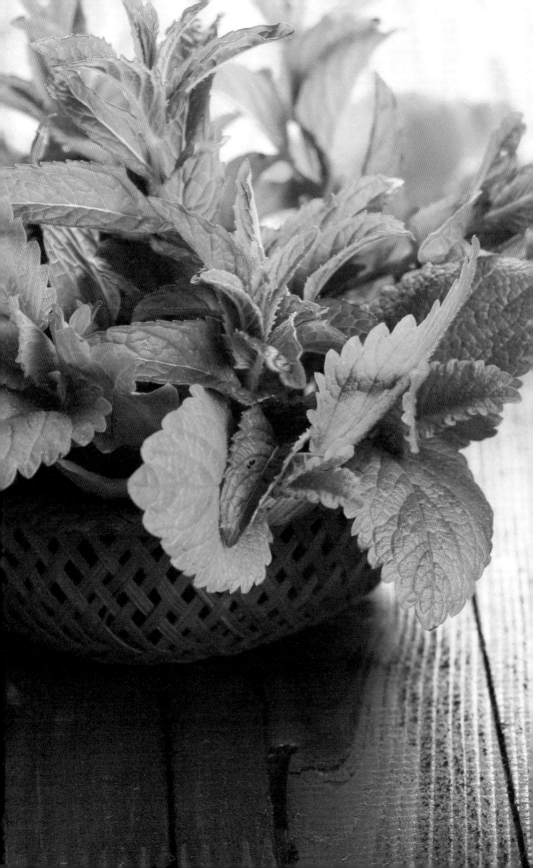

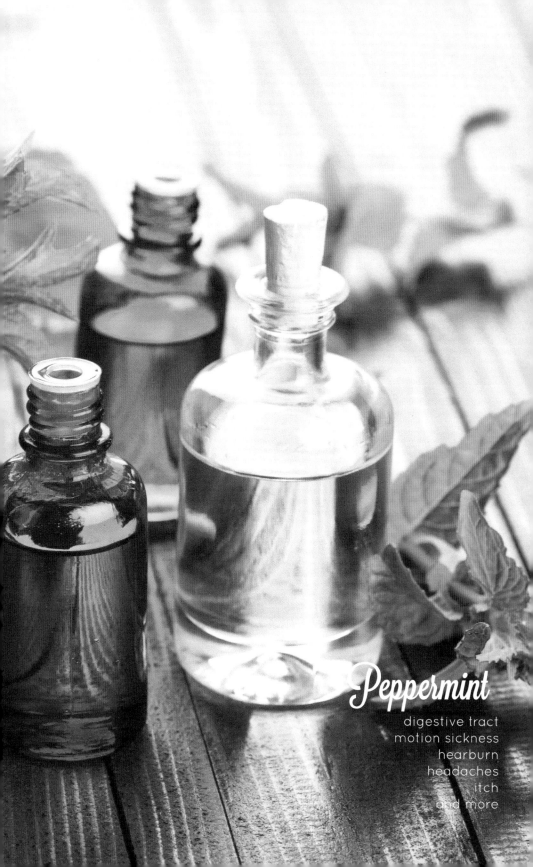

Peppermint

digestive tract
motion sickness
hearburn
headaches
itch
and more

Recipe Name:

Uses:

Family Results Record:

Date	Family Member	Condition	Application	Result

Recipe Name:

Uses:

Family Results Record:

Date	Family Member	Condition	Application	Result

Recipe Name:

Uses:

Family Results Record:

Date	Family Member	Condition	Application	Result

Recipe Name:

Uses:

Family Results Record:

Date	Family Member	Condition	Application	Result

Recipe Name:

Uses:

Family Results Record:

Date	Family Member	Condition	Application	Result

Recipe Name:

Uses:

Family Results Record:

Date	Family Member	Condition	Application	Result

Recipe Name:

Uses:

Family Results Record:

Date	Family Member	Condition	Application	Result

Recipe Name:

Uses:

Family Results Record:

Date	Family Member	Condition	Application	Result

Recipe Name:

Uses:

Family Results Record:

Date	Family Member	Condition	Application	Result

Recipe Name:

Uses:

Family Results Record:

Date	Family Member	Condition	Application	Result

Recipe Name:

Uses:

Family Results Record:

Date	Family Member	Condition	Application	Result

Recipe Name:

Uses:

Family Results Record:

Date	Family Member	Condition	Application	Result

Recipe Name:

Uses:

Family Results Record:

Date	Family Member	Condition	Application	Result

Recipe Name:

Uses:

Family Results Record:

Date	Family Member	Condition	Application	Result

Recipe Name:

Uses:

Family Results Record:

Date	Family Member	Condition	Application	Result

Recipe Name:

Uses:

Family Results Record:

Date	Family Member	Condition	Application	Result

Recipe Name:

Uses:

Family Results Record:

Date	Family Member	Condition	Application	Result

Recipe Name:

Uses:

Family Results Record:

Date	Family Member	Condition	Application	Result

Recipe Name:

Uses:

Family Results Record:

Date	Family Member	Condition	Application	Result

Recipe Name:

Uses:

Family Results Record:

Date	Family Member	Condition	Application	Result

Recipe Name:

Uses:

Family Results Record:

Date	Family Member	Condition	Application	Result

Recipe Name:

Uses:

Family Results Record:

Date	Family Member	Condition	Application	Result

Recipe Name:

Uses:

Family Results Record:

Date	Family Member	Condition	Application	Result

Recipe Name:

Uses:

Family Results Record:

Date	Family Member	Condition	Application	Result

Recipe Name:

Uses:

Family Results Record:

Date	Family Member	Condition	Application	Result

Recipe Name:

Uses:

Family Results Record:

Date	Family Member	Condition	Application	Result

Recipe Name:

Uses:

Family Results Record:

Date	Family Member	Condition	Application	Result

Recipe Name:

Uses:

Family Results Record:

Date	Family Member	Condition	Application	Result

Recipe Name:

Uses:

Family Results Record:

Date	Family Member	Condition	Application	Result

Recipe Name:

Uses:

Family Results Record:

Date	Family Member	Condition	Application	Result

Recipe Name:

Uses:

Family Results Record:

Date	Family Member	Condition	Application	Result

Recipe Name:

Uses:

Family Results Record:

Date	Family Member	Condition	Application	Result

Recipe Name:

Uses:

Family Results Record:

Date	Family Member	Condition	Application	Result

Recipe Name:

Uses:

Family Results Record:

Date	Family Member	Condition	Application	Result

Recipe Name:

Uses:

Family Results Record:

Date	Family Member	Condition	Application	Result

Recipe Name:

Uses:

Family Results Record:

Date	Family Member	Condition	Application	Result

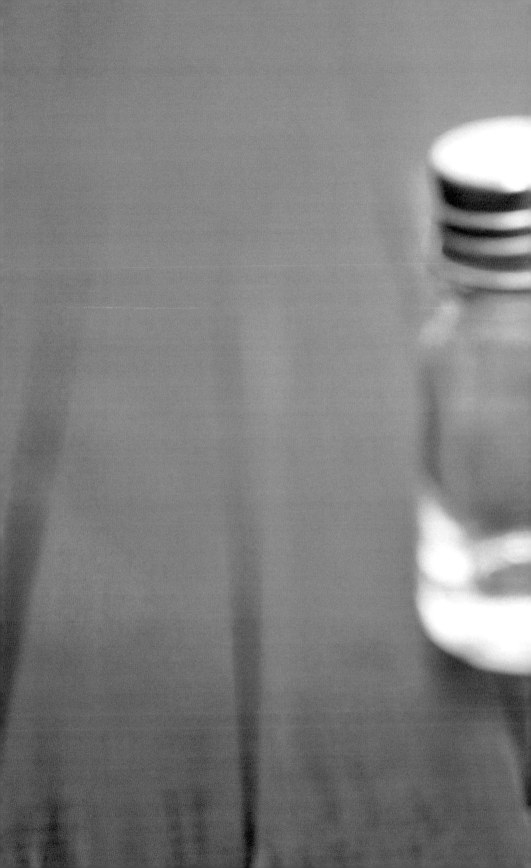

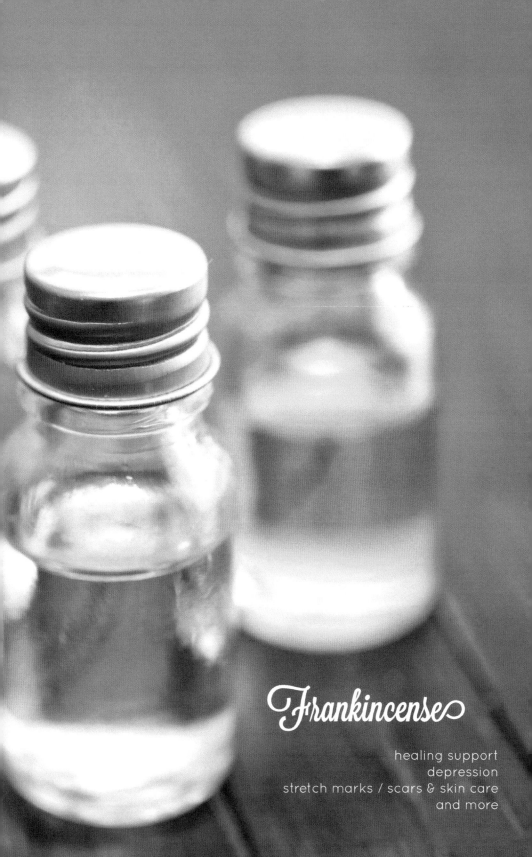

Frankincense

healing support
depression
stretch marks / scars & skin care
and more

Recipe Name:

Uses:

Family Results Record:

Date	Family Member	Condition	Application	Result

Recipe Name:

Uses:

Family Results Record:

Date	Family Member	Condition	Application	Result

Recipe Name:

_____

Uses:

_____

_____

_____

_____

Family Results Record:

Date	Family Member	Condition	Application	Result

Recipe Name:

_____

Uses:

_____

_____

_____

_____

Family Results Record:

Date	Family Member	Condition	Application	Result

Recipe Name:

Uses:

Family Results Record:

Date	Family Member	Condition	Application	Result

Recipe Name:

Uses:

Family Results Record:

Date	Family Member	Condition	Application	Result

Recipe Name:

Uses:

Family Results Record:

Date	Family Member	Condition	Application	Result

Recipe Name:

Uses:

Family Results Record:

Date	Family Member	Condition	Application	Result

Recipe Name:

Uses:

Family Results Record:

Date	Family Member	Condition	Application	Result

Recipe Name:

Uses:

Family Results Record:

Date	Family Member	Condition	Application	Result

Recipe Name:

Uses:

Family Results Record:

Date	Family Member	Condition	Application	Result

Recipe Name:

Uses:

Family Results Record:

Date	Family Member	Condition	Application	Result

Recipe Name:

Uses:

Family Results Record:

Date	Family Member	Condition	Application	Result

Recipe Name:

Uses:

Family Results Record:

Date	Family Member	Condition	Application	Result

Recipe Name:

Uses:

Family Results Record:

Date	Family Member	Condition	Application	Result

Recipe Name:

Uses:

Family Results Record:

Date	Family Member	Condition	Application	Result

Recipe Name:

Uses:

Family Results Record:

Date	Family Member	Condition	Application	Result

Recipe Name:

Uses:

Family Results Record:

Date	Family Member	Condition	Application	Result

Recipe Name:

Uses:

Family Results Record:

Date	Family Member	Condition	Application	Result

Recipe Name:

Uses:

Family Results Record:

Date	Family Member	Condition	Application	Result

Recipe Name:

Uses:

Family Results Record:

Date	Family Member	Condition	Application	Result

Recipe Name:

Uses:

Family Results Record:

Date	Family Member	Condition	Application	Result

Recipe Name:

Uses:

Family Results Record:

Date	Family Member	Condition	Application	Result

Recipe Name:

Uses:

Family Results Record:

Date	Family Member	Condition	Application	Result

Recipe Name:

Uses:

Family Results Record:

Date	Family Member	Condition	Application	Result

Recipe Name:

Uses:

Family Results Record:

Date	Family Member	Condition	Application	Result

Recipe Name:

Uses:

Family Results Record:

Date	Family Member	Condition	Application	Result

Recipe Name:

Uses:

Family Results Record:

Date	Family Member	Condition	Application	Result

Recipe Name:

Uses:

Family Results Record:

Date	Family Member	Condition	Application	Result

Recipe Name:

Uses:

Family Results Record:

Date	Family Member	Condition	Application	Result

Recipe Name:

Uses:

Family Results Record:

Date	Family Member	Condition	Application	Result

Recipe Name:

Uses:

Family Results Record:

Date	Family Member	Condition	Application	Result

Recipe Name:

Uses:

Family Results Record:

Date	Family Member	Condition	Application	Result

Recipe Name:

Uses:

Family Results Record:

Date	Family Member	Condition	Application	Result

Recipe Name:

Uses:

Family Results Record:

Date	Family Member	Condition	Application	Result

Recipe Name:

Uses:

Family Results Record:

Date	Family Member	Condition	Application	Result

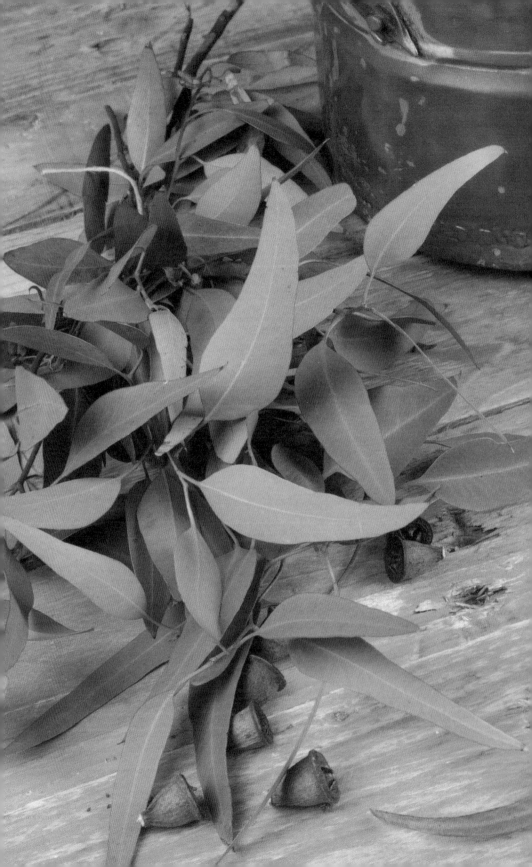

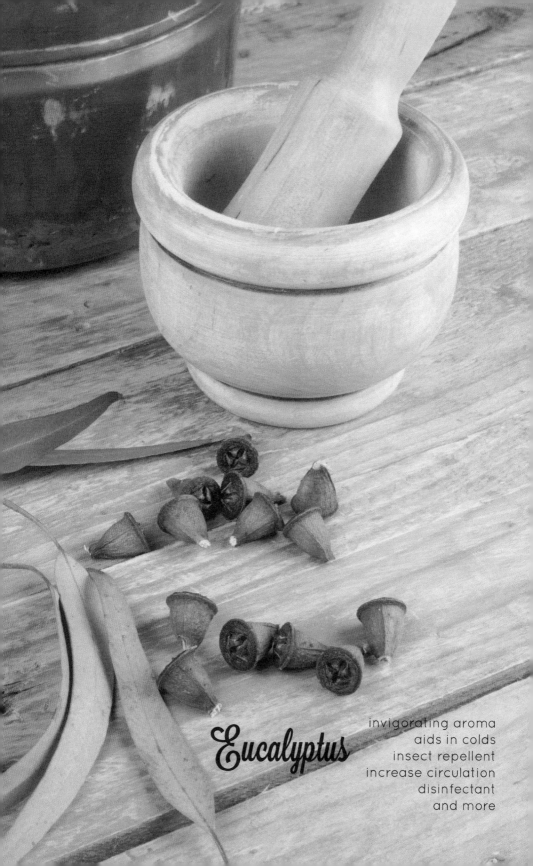

Eucalyptus

invigorating aroma
aids in colds
insect repellent
increase circulation
disinfectant
and more

Recipe Name:

Uses:

Family Results Record:

Date	Family Member	Condition	Application	Result

Recipe Name:

Uses:

Family Results Record:

Date	Family Member	Condition	Application	Result

Recipe Name:

Uses:

Family Results Record:

Date	Family Member	Condition	Application	Result

Recipe Name:

Uses:

Family Results Record:

Date	Family Member	Condition	Application	Result

Recipe Name:

Uses:

Family Results Record:

Date	Family Member	Condition	Application	Result

Recipe Name:

Uses:

Family Results Record:

Date	Family Member	Condition	Application	Result

Recipe Name:

Uses:

Family Results Record:

Date	Family Member	Condition	Application	Result

Recipe Name:

Uses:

Family Results Record:

Date	Family Member	Condition	Application	Result

Recipe Name:

Uses:

Family Results Record:

Date	Family Member	Condition	Application	Result

Recipe Name:

Uses:

Family Results Record:

Date	Family Member	Condition	Application	Result

Recipe Name:

Uses:

Family Results Record:

Date	Family Member	Condition	Application	Result

Recipe Name:

Uses:

Family Results Record:

Date	Family Member	Condition	Application	Result

Recipe Name:

Uses:

Family Results Record:

Date	Family Member	Condition	Application	Result

Recipe Name:

Uses:

Family Results Record:

Date	Family Member	Condition	Application	Result

Recipe Name:

Uses:

Family Results Record:

Date	Family Member	Condition	Application	Result

Recipe Name:

Uses:

Family Results Record:

Date	Family Member	Condition	Application	Result

Recipe Name:

Uses:

Family Results Record:

Date	Family Member	Condition	Application	Result

Recipe Name:

Uses:

Family Results Record:

Date	Family Member	Condition	Application	Result

Recipe Name:

Uses:

Family Results Record:

Date	Family Member	Condition	Application	Result

Recipe Name:

Uses:

Family Results Record:

Date	Family Member	Condition	Application	Result

Recipe Name:

Uses:

Family Results Record:

Date	Family Member	Condition	Application	Result

Recipe Name:

Uses:

Family Results Record:

Date	Family Member	Condition	Application	Result

Recipe Name:

Uses:

Family Results Record:

Date	Family Member	Condition	Application	Result

Recipe Name:

Uses:

Family Results Record:

Date	Family Member	Condition	Application	Result

Recipe Name:

Uses:

Family Results Record:

Date	Family Member	Condition	Application	Result

Recipe Name:

Uses:

Family Results Record:

Date	Family Member	Condition	Application	Result

Recipe Name:

Uses:

Family Results Record:

Date	Family Member	Condition	Application	Result

Recipe Name:

Uses:

Family Results Record:

Date	Family Member	Condition	Application	Result

Recipe Name:

Uses:

Family Results Record:

Date	Family Member	Condition	Application	Result

Recipe Name:

Uses:

Family Results Record:

Date	Family Member	Condition	Application	Result

Recipe Name:

Uses:

Family Results Record:

Date	Family Member	Condition	Application	Result

Recipe Name:

Uses:

Family Results Record:

Date	Family Member	Condition	Application	Result

Recipe Name: ෆ⚗ 🙍

Uses:

Family Results Record:

Date	Family Member	Condition	Application	Result

Recipe Name: ෆ⚗ 🙍

Uses:

Family Results Record:

Date	Family Member	Condition	Application	Result

Recipe Name:

Uses:

Family Results Record:

Date	Family Member	Condition	Application	Result

Recipe Name:

Uses:

Family Results Record:

Date	Family Member	Condition	Application	Result

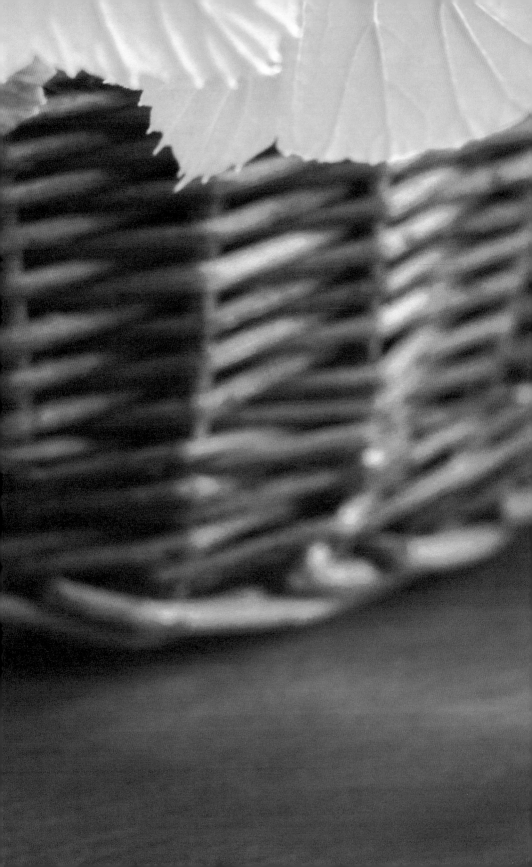

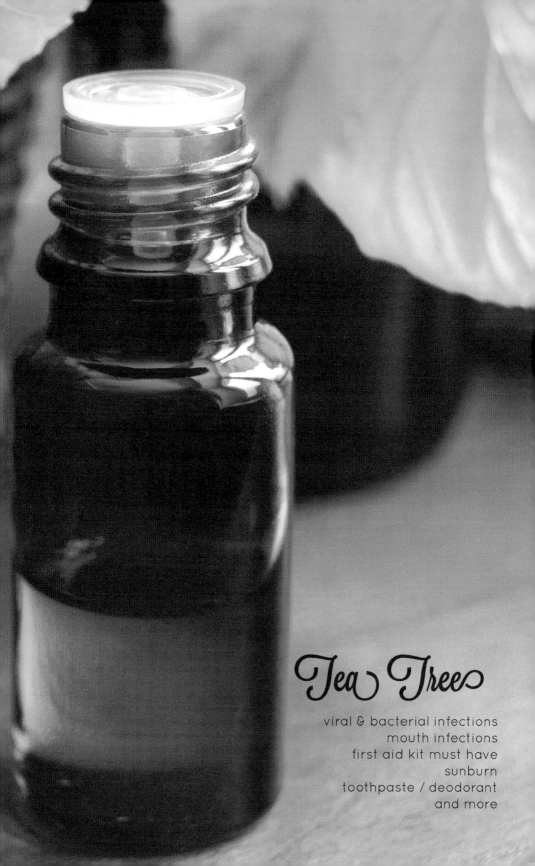

Tea Tree

viral & bacterial infections
mouth infections
first aid kit must have
sunburn
toothpaste / deodorant
and more

Recipe Name:

Uses:

Family Results Record:

Date	Family Member	Condition	Application	Result

Recipe Name:

Uses:

Family Results Record:

Date	Family Member	Condition	Application	Result

Recipe Name:

Uses:

Family Results Record:

Date	Family Member	Condition	Application	Result

Recipe Name:

Uses:

Family Results Record:

Date	Family Member	Condition	Application	Result

Recipe Name:

Uses:

Family Results Record:

Date	Family Member	Condition	Application	Result

Recipe Name:

Uses:

Family Results Record:

Date	Family Member	Condition	Application	Result

Recipe Name:

Uses:

Family Results Record:

Date	Family Member	Condition	Application	Result

Recipe Name:

Uses:

Family Results Record:

Date	Family Member	Condition	Application	Result

Recipe Name:

Uses:

Family Results Record:

Date	Family Member	Condition	Application	Result

Recipe Name:

Uses:

Family Results Record:

Date	Family Member	Condition	Application	Result

Recipe Name:

Uses:

Family Results Record:

Date	Family Member	Condition	Application	Result

Recipe Name:

Uses:

Family Results Record:

Date	Family Member	Condition	Application	Result

Recipe Name:

Uses:

Family Results Record:

Date	Family Member	Condition	Application	Result

Recipe Name:

Uses:

Family Results Record:

Date	Family Member	Condition	Application	Result

Recipe Name:

Uses:

Family Results Record:

Date	Family Member	Condition	Application	Result

Recipe Name:

Uses:

Family Results Record:

Date	Family Member	Condition	Application	Result

Recipe Name:

Uses:

Family Results Record:

Date	Family Member	Condition	Application	Result

Recipe Name:

Uses:

Family Results Record:

Date	Family Member	Condition	Application	Result

Recipe Name:

Uses:

Family Results Record:

Date	Family Member	Condition	Application	Result

Recipe Name:

Uses:

Family Results Record:

Date	Family Member	Condition	Application	Result

Recipe Name:

Uses:

Family Results Record:

Date	Family Member	Condition	Application	Result

Recipe Name:

Uses:

Family Results Record:

Date	Family Member	Condition	Application	Result

Recipe Name:

Uses:

Family Results Record:

Date	Family Member	Condition	Application	Result

Recipe Name:

Uses:

Family Results Record:

Date	Family Member	Condition	Application	Result

Recipe Name:

Uses:

Family Results Record:

Date	Family Member	Condition	Application	Result

Recipe Name:

Uses:

Family Results Record:

Date	Family Member	Condition	Application	Result

Recipe Name:

Uses:

Family Results Record:

Date	Family Member	Condition	Application	Result

Recipe Name:

Uses:

Family Results Record:

Date	Family Member	Condition	Application	Result

My Essential Oil Stock

☐	Angelica	
☐	Basil	
☐	Bergamot	
☐	Black Pepper	
☐	Blue Cypress	
☐	Blue Tansy	
☐	Cardamom	
☐	Carrot Seed	
☐	Cedarwood	
☐	Celery Seed	
☐	Cinnamon Bark	
☐	Cistus	
☐	Citronella	
☐	Clary Sage	
☐	Clove	
☐	Copaiba	
☐	Coriander	
☐	Cypress	
☐	Dill	
☐	Dorado Azul	
☐	Elemi	
☐	Eucalyptus Blue	
☐	Eucalyptus Globulus	
☐	Eucalyptus Radiata	
☐	Fennel	
☐	Frankincense	
☐	Galbanum	
☐	German Chamomile	
☐	Ginger	
☐	Goldenrod	
☐	Grapefruit	
☐	Helichrysum	
☐	Hinoki	
☐	Hyssop	
☐	Idaho Balsam Fir	

☐	Idaho Blue Spruce	
☐	Idaho Tansy	
☐	Jasmine	
☐	Juniper	
☐	Laurus Nobilis	
☐	Lavender	
☐	Ledum	
☐	Lemon	
☐	Lemongrass	
☐	Lemon Myrtle	
☐	Lime	
☐	Marjoram	
☐	Melaleuca Alternifolia	
☐	Melaleuca Ericifolia	
☐	Melaleuca Quinquenervia	
☐	Melissa	
☐	Mountain Savory	
☐	Myrrh	
☐	Myrtle	
☐	Neroli	
☐	Nutmeg	
☐	Ocotea	
☐	Orange	
☐	Oregano	
☐	Palmarosa	
☐	Palo Santo	
☐	Patchouli	
☐	Peppermint	
☐	Petitgrain	
☐	Pine	
☐	Ravintsara	
☐	Roman Chamomile	
☐	Rose	
☐	Rosemary	
☐	Sacred Frankincense	
☐	Sacred Frankincense	
☐	Sage	

☐	Sandalwood	
☐	Spearmint	
☐	Spikenard	
☐	St. Maries Lavender	
☐	Tangerine	
☐	Tarragon	
☐	Thyme	
☐	Tsuga	
☐	Valerian	
☐	Vetiver	
☐	Western Red Cedar	
☐	Wintergreen	
☐	Ylang Ylang	
☐		
☐		
☐		
☐		
☐		
☐		
☐		
☐		
☐		
☐		
☐		
☐		
☐		
☐		
☐		
☐		
☐		
☐		
☐		
☐		
☐		
☐		
☐		

41762958R00085

Made in the USA
Lexington, KY
26 May 2015